Reflexology: A Beginners Guide To

Reflexology

Learn Easy Massage Techniques To Relieve Foot Pain And Reduce Stress

By

Michele Gilbert

Visit Amazon's Michele Gilbert Page

Dedicated to those who choose to stretch beyond their own limits

And to seek a more abundant and fulfilling life.

Your thoughts are creative.

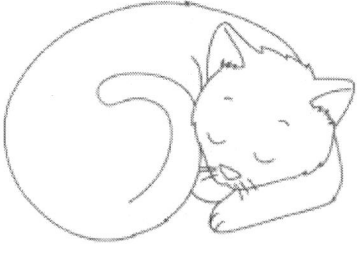

Michele Gilbert

<<< My Free Gift For You>>>

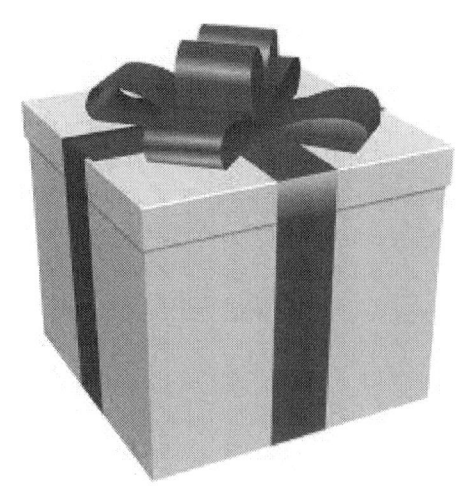

Introduction

Have you ever had a really good massage? It's not something that you can easily forget. Honestly, if you've had a really long, hard day, the one thing that you're going to really want to enjoy is to take off your shoes and have a really great foot massage. How about writing a really long book report or anything where you're writing a whole bunch? You want to have a massage, get the muscles relaxed and get them all happy again after a lot of hard work you probably didn't want to do anyways. It's fantastic. Massages have the ability to make everything great again. Seriously, a massage has therapeutic powers.

Of course, we might think that it's a funny joke or an amusing thought that kind of just passes through your head while you're enjoying some serious massage actions. There is a power in the massage out there that is more than just a way of relaxing but actually taking care of your body. It's the kind of miraculous power over the human body that eventually led people to wonder what other powers the human body is capable of with just the ability of human touch.

    The human touch is something that has held the power and sway over many medical professionals, spiritualists, and holy individuals all around the world who have benefited contact with the hurting, injured, or sick as healing them. It's this power that has drawn attention to a particular skill and power that practitioners have honed and mastered over the centuries that is popping up all around the world today. It's known as reflexology and it's the art of using touch to cure people of their aches, their pains, and getting people back into their lives without sacrificing anything more than they already have for the agony in their life.

Reflexology is a growing field that is full of mystery and might not be what most people would think it is. Specifically, people probably look at the word reflexology and think that I'm trying to teach you the science of catching something your kids throw at your head. Well, it has nothing to do about your reflexes really, but it does have something to do with something called reflex zones. This is all, of course, just a taste for you. I'm whetting your appetite for what's to come.

It's a fascinating subject. It's something that will really intrigue you and grab your attention. So, in this book, I'm going to show you what reflexology is, how you can participate with it in your life, and all the information that you're going to need to know. It's going to be the best introduction to reflexology that you could possibly find. So sit back and get comfortable. You're about to learn what it means to be a practitioner of reflexology and how that's going to radically change the way you enjoy your life.

So let's get started!

What Is Reflexology?

So, I know what you're thinking. What is reflexology and why is it a thing? Some of you might also be thinking about something a little deeper, such as: how is this applicable, how do I get started, what is the history, or something along those lines. Well, the answers are going to make you think about what reflexology is and how you're going to be able to handle it in your life. In the end, reflexology is one of those skills that the deeper you look into it, the more you're going to want to gain experience and practice it. It's going to be great.

The history of reflexology is fairly broad and fairly extensive. What it comes down to is the fact that there is a lot history that is loaded with the application of physical touch to make people cope with their suffering, whether physical, mental, or spiritual. I'm going to hit the history of all of these. It's something that is really hard to escape.

One really doesn't have to look much farther than the extensive history of eastern medicine to see just how far back the application of physical touch has been in the use of physicians. Whether you're looking at acupuncture or massage, there are focal points on the human body where pressure can cause pain to be released and euphoria to set in. This has been true since the first human rubbed a cramp out of their muscle and since then, physicians have been working on honing and applying this technique to their practices. There is evidence f this in ancient Egypt, China, and in North American tribes.

It wasn't until the modern era that people started putting a name to the idea that you could apply pressure on areas of your body that would influence the feeling of other parts. It was often joked that a person who had a toothache should squeeze their toe to get some relief from it. During the 16th century, the idea of Zone Therapy began to become more and more prominent. This idea, that there are zones in the bodies and that there are ways to access them from different places in the body became more and more popular and more and more time was dedicated to the research of it.

Mentally, there have been many attributes of massage and the care of the human body that has been linked to a better way of living. The idea of keeping stress and discomfort locked away in your body has a way of bogging down you psyche and there has been a lot of experimentation into the psychological aspects of Reflexology as well. The ability to relieve pressure and tension that has nestled its way deep into your nervous system, muscles, or joints, is something that you'll never want to lose and that you'll never give up. It's a power that so many people would love to have and it's easy for people to learn and apply easily. This makes it highly effective and people caught onto it a long time ago. That's why most people commonly will think of getting a massage whenever times are getting tough or things are getting harder in their life. Have a hard week at work and by Friday, you're thinking about going and getting a massage. It's that prominent in our culture.

    The final aspect, of the history of Reflexology, is the spiritual aspect of it, which is extremely common among cultures. I'd dare to say that beyond the physical and mental benefits of touch, the spiritual aspect is the most popular and excitable aspect of Reflexology. The spiritual side of using pressure or testing your body to have an enlightening experience and the laying on of hands has been a part of cultures all across the world. We want the presence of holy men and holy women laying on their hands and taking away pain and suffering. Whether you're a person who likes to pass your positive energy, show fellowship, or pass on wisdom, the ability to put your hands upon your friends and family, while being able to take care of them and remove some of the suffering and pain, then you'll want to hone and master it.

    The history of Reflexology is the history of human touch. It's extensive and it's prominent in the world of spiritual, mental, and physical well-being. It's the very history of our people and you're going to find that Reflexology is the culmination of everything that we've learned up to this point. So, are your ready to learn about bringing around the history of human touch and mastering it? Well, then let's get started.

The Basics of Reflexology

Reflexology really can be divided up into two sections of focus that people really tend to work towards when they're diving into the world of massage through relief. The two main places that the world comes in contact with and that's your hands and your feet. Sure, pressure points, muscle groups, and joints tend to play a role in the world of massage and relaxation, but for the basics of Reflexology, you're really going to find that the feet and the hands of the body are going to be the most important parts. The reason for this is simple and it's going to be easy for you to understand why you're going to want to focus on these two areas the most.

The hand is a clear choice when it comes to dealing with the aspects of Reflexology. If you take a moment to think about your hands, you're actually going to be blown away by just what it is exactly that your hands mean to your body. Your hands are the workers of the body. They are going to help you maintain your body and the world around you. Without your hands, your life becomes infinitely much harder, but that doesn't make it impossible. It just makes it difficult. With our hands, we feed and hydrate ourselves, shelter and clothe ourselves, and most importantly, we entertain ourselves with our hands. All work is done with the palms, fingers, and thumbs, without any of them, it's so hard. With that simple realization, everything that you bring on in your life or everything that you encounter, you're probably going to touch it, work with it, or try to get rid of it with your hands. This means that they're the point of conflict, tension, stress, and purpose in our lives. They are the key to our survival and our success. So, when your body isn't feeling well, there's a good possibility that it's entered through the hands and that means there's a way to deal with it using your hands.

The second point of the body that is going to be of extreme focus, like I've mentioned before, is the feet. Now, unlike the hands, our feet are not the point of conflict and contact with most of the things in our life, rather, they are the transportation that we use to retreat and approach things. If we need something and cannot reach out and take it with our hands, then our feet are going to have to do the job for us. That means that our feet are what take us to the events we encounter within our lives. Our feet take us to our happiest moments and our darkest days, without them, we are stagnant beings with nothing new or different in our lives. With that being said, you carry a lot of stress and a lot of burdens through your body and it can all bottle up in your feet. That's why Reflexology tends to focus the majority of its time on your feet as well as your hands.

    So, feet and hands, those are the two big points in Reflexology. This is going to be where the majority of your focus is going to be when you're working on relieving pain throughout the body. I'm not talking about using some massage techniques to relieve pain in your feet and hands. I'm talking about back pain, stomach pain, and any kind of pain that you could think of that is bothering you the most. We are linked everywhere and we are entirely capable of relieving yourself of the pain that plagues you or the people you know.

This is something that you can learn and harness for yourself. Now that we know the two basics, then let's have a look at the skills you can put to work on the feet.

The Basics of the Foot

Now, as we've already discussed, your feet have amazing properties that the rest of your body really doesn't possess. There's something about the feet that make us people of adventure, work, and society. It's something very few of us realize until it's pointed out to us and that means that there's something truly powerful about our feet. It also makes them a focal point to the practitioners of Reflexology. Your feet are attached to all over your body and you're going to find that there's a whole lot of technique, style, and knowledge that comes to your feet. There's an entire map of your feet which shows how you're going to access your entire body simply by massaging your feet. It's an incredible map and I'm going to give you a brief overview of each of them.

I'm going to start with the bottom of your feet. It's the largest chunk of the foot that we're going to be examining. It can be divided four sections and then I'll be going in deeper and more intimately into the sections of the foot for you to fully understand what each section means. So, with each section, I'll go over the basics and then we'll dive in deeper before moving on.

Starting off, the first section that we're going to look at are the toes. Your toes are actually quite fascinating for what exactly it is that you can do with them and what it is that they're connected to. Remember how I gave the example of the old saying where if you have a toothache, you rub your big toe? Well, there's a lot of evidence pointing to that. Your toes are the first major section and strangely enough, there are strong links to the head and neck. It's not just the head and neck in a vague term, but it's also the fact that if you have everything from muscle pain to migraines or even sinus pressure, you're going to find a cure to that with your toes. There's plenty areas that you're going to want to explores, so you're going to find it delightful when I start to show you these fascinating things.

The tops of your toes are going to be the places that you'll probably find yourself exploring the most. The tops of your toes are fascinating and they're quite extensive. When you experiment with the pain of your head and neck, you'll find that each toe reacts differently to your pain. If you have aching pain in your tooth, sinus pressure or pain, or even if you have pain on the top of your head, then you're going to want to deal with the toes. These are all going to be dealt with at the tips of your toes where you can massage until you feel the pain subsiding. I usually start with the big toe and then keep working until I find the link that helps the most. Apply pressure and massage gently until the pain is gone.

    The middle of your pinky toe and the preceding toe, you're going to find that you are able to work out ear pain. If the middle joint of your toe isn't doing the trick, work the area between the two toes and the pads of the muscles until you find the sweet spot. The next following pair of toes are where you're going to find relief for you eyes, especially if you're feeling pressure or dizziness from a headache or just looking at a screen for too long. Massage these points and get the most out of it.

The section I'm going to discuss next is the pads of your feet. This is going to be the muscle group that exists between your toes and the arch of your feet. This area is really specifically targeted toward your chests and the organs within your torso that are going to help you. If there is any kind of trouble or pain or illness that you're experiencing inside your chest, this is going to be where it is you're going to be focusing your time. It's something that you're going to find yourself working with more and more. So, let's see what you can really get done when you are working over your feet.

The ball of muscle right under your big toe is where you're going to find some incredibly relief for glands all over your body. Everything is going to start working better and better with the glands all over your body as you massage this part of your foot. You're going to notice that swollen glands or enlarged glands are going to really start to relax and stop being inflamed. The next area toward the center of your foot is where you're going to focus if you have any kind of congestion or difficult breathing. It's going to strengthen your lungs and it's going to clear out your respiratory system. You'll find that breathing becomes easier and clearer. Finally, deep in the center of your foot, almost to the arch, that sweet spot between the arch and the muscular area, you'll find that this is the place for your heart. This is often a spiritual aspect where people use them to build up courage, love, and strength.

Next, let's talk about the arch of your foot. This is going to be the area from fleshy, muscly part of your foot that stretches all the way down to the heel of your foot. This extension of your arch is a place where you're going to find a whole lot of work that you can do with your body. You're going to find a lot of organ work available to you as well. Your waist and abdomen are going to be the core focus of this point of your foot. There's a lot of places that you can find access in this portion of your foot and I'm going to give you a look at all of it. We're going to start from the interior of your foot as well and work our way out.

    At the top of your left arch, just under the pads of your feet, you're going to find an access point to your stomach to help with digestion, cramping, or any other pain that you might be suffering. Working your way across to the outside of your foot, you're going to find an access point for your spleen. For your right foot, rather than the stomach and spleen, you'll be accessing your liver. Right under this area at the interior of your foot, you're going to find access points to your pancreas and kidneys on both of your feet. Now, at the heart of your arch, near the bottom, you're going to find that you'll have access to your small intestines, but the surrounding area is where you'll find access to your large intestines. This is going to really help you work with digestion and make it so that you can have smooth bowel movements.

    The final aspect of the bottom of your foot is the heel and this is a section that is specifically created for the pelvic area and you'll also find that there's something attached to relieving pain in your legs. This is really a simple and basic area and that means that you're not going to find a whole lot of diversity in this area. Essentially, a band that goes right over the center of your heel to work your sciatic nerve. This is going to relieve a lot of pain, especially if you have sciatic troubles. This essentially concludes the bottom of your foot.

Now, let's have a chat about the inside of your foot. This is where you're going to find a lot of more effective areas to help heal whatever aches you. The bottom of the inside of your foot is a band that you're going to want to work to help alleviate spine and back problems that you might be suffering from. The center of your arch, you're going to find a portion of your foot to massage where you'll relieve bladder pain that you might be suffering from.

Moving over to the top of your foot, you're going to find that the top of your foot is mostly tied to the muscular pain of your chest, rather than the organ based relief that you'll find on the bottom of your feet. Moving back toward your ankle on the top of your foot, you'll find that this is more focused on the health and maintenance of your lymphatic system. When you've reached the actual base of your foot and your ankle, you'll find that this area is focused on the health of your groin area. This is where you'll really start to work all the pain that you might be suffering from a pulled groin muscle. If you've ever suffered from a pulled groin, then you'll know how valuable it'll be to have this exercise to help heal what aches you.

Now, the outside of the foot, I'm going to start just below your pinky toe. Right here, that area on the side of the muscular ball, this area is going to where you're going to want to focus when you're looking to relieve any pain that you are suffering from in your shoulders. Below that, you're going to find the outside of your arch, which is going to really help you with any elbow pain that you might be suffering from. This is a spot to focus on for anyone that is really effective with those of you who play sports. At the base of your arch on the outside of your foot, you're going to find that we're transitioning to your legs. This section is going to focus on your hips and keeping pain at bay. Below that on the ball of your foot, you'll find that this area is tied to your knee pain that you might be suffering from.

  This wraps up the areas of your foot that you can work to help heal the pains in your body just from massaging your foot. There are plenty of actual massaging techniques that will help you target and really get to the pain you're suffering from, but there's more to work with on your hands, which we'll talk about in the next chapter. Remember to really get creative and look up the best massage techniques that are going to help you really get the most out of your massage. With this knowledge, you'll be able to really get to work on your feet. Next up, let's have a look at your hands.

The Basics of the Hands

As I talked about earlier, you're going to find that your hands actually play a huge role in your life. This is where you come in contact with the world all around you. This is where you want to go when you're actually suffering from physical pain. This is what you're looking for when you're encountering pain that you've brought upon yourself through the interaction of the life around you and the change that you're trying to implement into your world around you. With the hands being very similar to the feet, you're going to really want to work both your hands and your feet to get the maximum results of your efforts.

When it comes to your hands, you're going to be mainly focusing on the bottoms of your hands. That means, if you're looking at the back of your hands, then you're looking at the wrong spot, so flip them over and take a look. When you're staring at your palms, then I want to direct your eyes to the bottoms of your palms and where your hands meets your wrists. This is going to be where I'm going to start focusing my discussion. I'll work from the bottom of your hand to the tips of your fingers and I'll go from the outside of your hand to the inside of your hand. Now, let's get to work.

At the bottom of your hands, you're going to find that this is the area of your hand where you want to physically and spiritually heal your genitalia. That's right, your junk is right at the bottom of your hand. With this, you'll need to massage and work it over to really become comfortable. Above that on the outside, you're going to find the area where you can really loosen up your shoulders and release the pain and tension that we all tend to carry in that area. Working your way inside, you'll find that right above the genitalia area, you're going to work an area to cure bladder pain and suffering you might be experiencing. Really focus on the bottom of that fleshy pad extending from the bottom of your thumb. Right at the base of that is where you're going to find your bladder point. Finally, the inside of that pad, along the edge of your hand, that's going to help you with spine tension and pain in your back.

    Focusing on the palm of your hand, you're going to find that on the outside of your hand, along the length of the exterior where your shoulder area is, just inside of that, you'll find the section for your heart. Like with your feet, the heart section is a very spiritual center, helping you exercise and open up the love, courage, and compassion that you're seeking in your life. Moving over to the heart of your palm, you're going to find two points, one right above the other. The top point, focused directly in the heart of your palm, this is your colon point. Massage this area to really relax the colon and help stimulate proper digestion. This is going to give you the digestion you're looking for. Just below that, where the valley of the palm and the pad of your thumb meet, that's the second point, which is where you'll massage to work your small intestines. Massage this area to help relax digestion pain and agony that you might be suffering from. Finally, next to that, on the inside of your hand where your thumb meets your palm, this is the area that links your hand to your stomach. Massage this area for ulcers, indigestion, constipation, or any kind of digestion issue that might be plaguing you. Finally, across the pads of your palm, at the base of your fingers, this is going to really open up your abdomen muscles and your hips, giving you the freedom to release the tension and pain that might be building in that area.

Finally, we're going to work the fingers and discuss the significance of each of them. Each finger is mostly identical until we reach your fingertips. I want you to look down at your fingers. All four of your fingers are divided up into three sections. There are your fingertips, the central section, and the base section. I'm going to start from the bottom and work my way up to your fingertips. If you think I've forgotten your thumb, then don't worry, I'll be hitting that in its own paragraph, so fear not!

Starting from the base section, right where your fingers meet the pads of your palm's top, you'll find that this are is really focused on your lungs and the respiration that you're bringing air into your life. Massage this area to help with any lung suffering you might be having. This is coughing or phlegm build up that you might be experiencing, not congestion or anything like that. Now, on the top of that base third, you'll find that the pinky and ring fingers are focused on ears. Massage this to relieve pressure, pain, or even hearing issues that you might be suffering from. With that same area in the middle and index finger, you'll find that this is focused on eye pain that you might be experiencing. Massage this area to help relieve pressure that is building up. For the central third of your fingers, this is where you're going to be focusing on your nasal and sinus passages. This is where you're going to want to focus if you're suffering from congestion, allergies, or pain from pressure build ups. Notice that your lungs and your sinuses each hit different areas and have vastly different purposes. Massage accordingly.

Now, when it comes to your fingertips, it's a completely different rodeo and each fingertip serves as a different point and a different focus to your body. So, each time you massage a fingertip, you'll be hitting a different area of your body. Starting with your pinky, this is the fingertip that you're going to want to hit if you're looking to work over you kidneys and your circulatory system. This is really going to help you with blood flow and getting the energy and nutrients you need to have distributed throughout your body done in a timely and effective manner. With your ring finger, you'll find that this is another area that really focuses on your lungs and you're breathing in general. If you're out of breath a lot or need to really focus on your breathing, try massaging your ring fingertip. As for your middle finger, this is where you're going to really work on your liver and oddly enough, your face. This is where you're going to stimulate wellness, balance, and an over all relaxed mentality. Your index finger is the point where you're going to want to touch on your stomach and digestive system. This is where you're in a crunch and really need to get some relief fast. This is the area that you'll really want to focus on.

Now, when it comes to your thumb, this is a digit that is really developed for the relief of muscle pain, particularly in your neck. When you're massaging your thumb, you're hitting a lot of levels that really come together in a harmony that promotes the best circumstances for your neck and throat. Starting from the base, you're hitting your thyroid and working your way up to your vocal chords. Whether you're doing this for physical or spiritual reasons, your vocal chords effect how you speak, how well your words come out, and how enduring your voice might be. Finally, the fleshy bad of your thumb, you'll be working the muscles of your neck and the wellness of your throat, helping you release all of that tension and stress that we build up in our necks. This is great for people who find themselves working in a desk environment all day long.

Your hands might seem very similar to your feet and there's a reason for that. Sometimes massaging your feet isn't enough and you need to really hit on some other tactics to release that deep tension and pain that has built up over time. Try both methods to get rid of the pain that is plaguing you. Now that you know the areas that you can work over on your hands and feet, I'm going to tell you that it's stupid to hit just one spot. I know, it kind of seems like a jerk move, but trust me, I have my reasons. Meet me in the next chapter and we'll talk all about it in detail.

The Massage

Now, I know what you're thinking. I just laid out a battle plan for you and I told you exactly where you need to target to really get that pain that's been bothering you for a long time out of your system and now I'm telling you not to target that area. Well, kind of—but not exactly.

In fact, what I'm saying is that Reflexology is a big picture and that kind of mentality is all about the small picture. If you're looking to get rid of the pain that's plaguing you, it's not just in one area. Pain is something that we've kind of gotten used to, which is a very sad and disappointing fact in the lives we live. In fact, we've gotten so tolerant to it that most of us have no clue that we're suffering and that we need relief. What Reflexology aims to do is to give your whole body a chance to scrub away the pain that has been lingering and hanging on like bad luggage for so long. This means not just focusing on one area, but hitting all of them.

Here's an example. Imagine you're in a sandbox and that you've decided to viciously and with fierce determination, to dig a hole in a single area. What happens to the sand? It starts to slip into the hole. Sure, it doesn't fill up entirely, but the sand comes back in that area. So too will the pain if you just hit one spot. That pain will come back, because you haven't eliminated all of it.

So, when giving a massage to yourself or another person, give them the relief that they need all over them. Even if you're just focusing on the abdomen, make sure that you hit the kidney, liver, stomach, intestines, and hips. Give them a full massage and not just a direct, strategic attack that isn't going to keep the pain away for long.

Secondly, remember that people who are hurting or who are suffering are often more prone to being sensitive and are not going to want extreme pressure. Be aware of this and don't treat them like a ball of dough that you need to knead into submission. Be gentle, be kind, and read their reactions that you're picking up on as you massage them.

Thirdly, start with the feet. I know that hands are much more comfortable because a lot of people in our world have issues with touching feet, but start out with a warm foot massage and then get to work gently massaging their feet, hitting those focal areas in a strategic manner so that the zones are nurtured and tended to. When you've hit their feet with a strong massage, then you can decided to move to their hands, but see first if you've helped them really relax and release some of that pain that they've been carrying with them.

    Finally, make sure that your subject is comfortable. This is often an overlooked sight for those that are first starting out, but make sure that they're at ease. This might be uncomfortable to you, but the more you massage someone, the more relaxed they become. This might mean abandoning your subject's feet and hands and really work the area to get that comfort level that you're looking for. Just as a word of warning, when people get relaxed, sometimes bodily functions happen. Be a professional and keep quiet about it. They don't need to hear how grossed out you are by the fact that they accidentally burped or passed gas.

As a word of warning, I know that Reflexology tends to get scooped up into the world of essential oils, creams, and lotions. From the experience that I've had and from the world that I've seen of Reflexology, you don't really need this. It's kind of an added ambient feature that people try very hard to tie in. If it helps you and it helps your client or subject, fine, use it. If it doesn't, then don't feel pressured into something that you're not comfortable with and make sure that it has a purpose. It's not magical and it's not going to miraculously make your technique any better. The only way your skill or technique is going to get better is with practice that you're going to have to dedicate your time to.

Essentially, get cracking on it and then see if all of the bells and whistles help you out in the end.

Conclusion

I hope that this book has been a big success for you. There have been a lot of people who are extremely interested in the subject of Reflexology and it kind of just looks like a glorified massage on the outside. While that's a fair guess, it's not quite hitting the heart of what Reflexology truly is. Through the promotion of wellness and balance, you'll find that Reflexology is a tool that you'll be using in your life for days to come. It has helped a lot of people and I'm sure it'll help you.

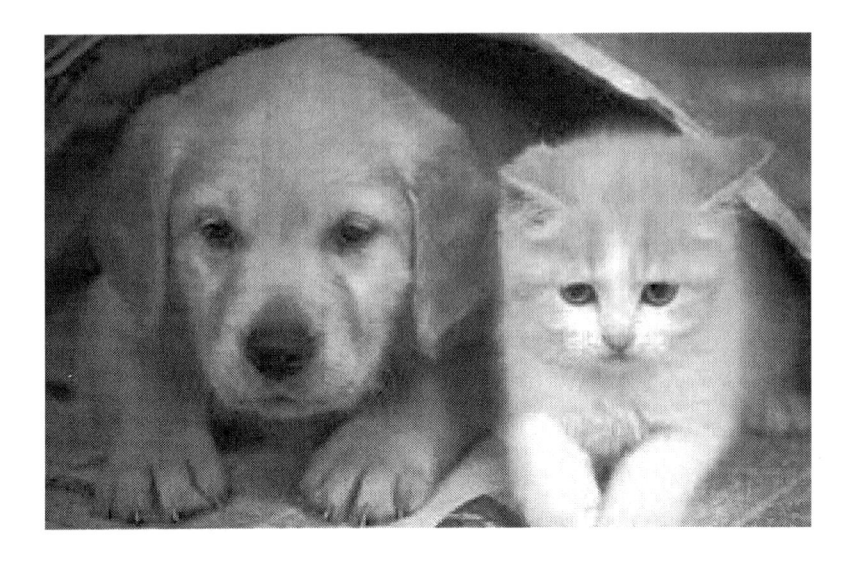

Before you go, I'd like to say thank you for purchasing my book.

I know you could have picked so many other books to read, but you took a chance on me.

So A Big thanks for downloading this book and reading it all the way to completion.

Now I would like to ask a *small* favor.

Could you please take a minute or two to leave a review for this book on Amazon?

Click here

The feedback will help me continue to publish more kindle books that will help people to get better results in their lives.

And if you found it helpful in anyway then please let me know :-)

My Free Gift To You!

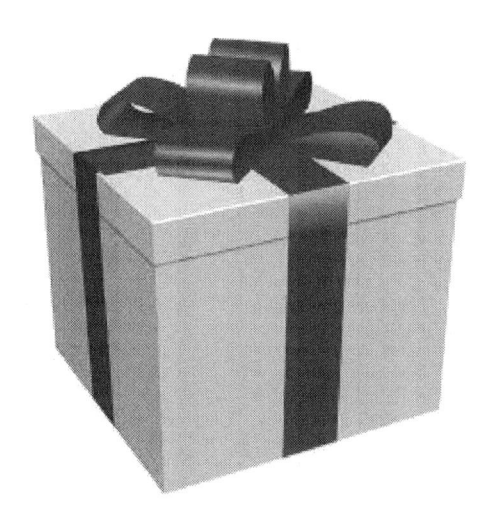

As a way of saying thank you for downloading my book, I am willing to give you access to a selected group of readers who (every week or so) receive inspiring, life-changing kindle books at deep discounts, and sometimes even absolutely free.

Wouldn't it be great to get amazing Kindle offers delivered directly to your inbox?

Wouldn't it be great to be the first to know when I'm releasing new fresh and above all sharply discounted content?

But why would I so something like this?

Why would I offer my books at such a low price and even give them away for free when they took me countless hours to produce?

Simple…. because I want to spread the word.!

For a few short days Amazon allows Kindle authors to promote their newly released books by offering them deeply discounted (up to 70% price discounts and even for free. This allows us to spread the word extremely quickly allowing users to download thousands and thousands of copies in a very short period of time.

Once the timeframe has passed, these books will revert back to their normal selling price. That's why you will benefit from being the first to know when they can be downloaded for free!

GET ACCESS NOW!

So are you ready to claim your weekly Kindle books?

You are just one click away! Follow the link below and sign up to start receiving awesome content

Thank you and Enjoy!

Preview of My New Book

[Tarot: Reading Tarot Cards: The Beginners Guidebook To The Ancient Art Of Tarot Card Meanings And Spreads](#)

What Do The Cards Say?

When it comes to Tarot Cards, it's hard not to think of cheesy scenes in movies or on TV shows that have really butchered and mocked the art of Tarot Cards to death. Fortunetellers are nothing more than Gypsy stereotypes that blatantly insult the Romani way of life and are the closest thing to racism that their culture has or can experience. But behind every enduring legend, there is something deeper that knocks on the door of our subconscious. What is it about Tarot Cards that makes us stop and linger outside of tents at fairs or festivals? What is it about those strange pictures that make us wonder if there is any real power behind them?

Want the simple answer?

You want there to be power.

Tarot Cards have been around for a long time and they have an irresistible and undeniable power on those that take the reading. Even those who consider themselves learned or the educated who are above such fabled superstitions cannot help but see that there is something powerful behind the cards, whether they want to admit it or not.

Today, I'm here to explain to you just what it is about Tarot cards that make them so unique and so powerful to people who sit through readings. I'll give you a brief history about what it is that has helped the cards endure and survive for so long and in the end, I'll give you a detailed understanding about each of the cards that will give you a basic understanding as to what they are and how you can utilize them in your basic readings.

I truly hope that you're ready to learn, because there is so much about Tarot Cards that you're going to learn and love to hear about. So let's not waste any more time and let's get to it.

A Brief History of Enchantment

Why are Tarot Cards so unique and so generally compelling? Because people think they're magical and they're anything but. The bitter truth that you might not want to hear is that there is nothing mystical and nothing supernatural about Tarot Cards. Now, instead of thinking of that as a negative, look at it through the lenses that I'm going to give you right now.

Tarot Cards are intimate, subconscious, psychological evaluations of the person coming to the table. Tarot Cards are unique and they're incredibly interesting and why the cards show up in the order that they do are quite entertaining for those of us who adopt the moniker of Reader. Essentially, when you display a card, you are giving them a Rorschach test that they're going to process and understand themselves. I'll go more into this later, but you'll come to understand that this is vital to your ability to actually give good readings.

As for Tarot Cards and their history, the idea has been around for a really long time and can honestly be traced back to Nordic Runes that were used to predict the outcomes and the events that were going to happen or even discern the answers to the questions that the caster asks. This idea of deriving understanding and wisdom from inanimate objects is known as divination and it has been around since civilization has existed. Primitive cultures even used the bones of dead animals, seashells, and even blood as a way of divining guidance from celestial beings. As society developed, the arts of divination were more refined and more manicured to fit the time period.

Click Here To Read More

Tarot: Reading Tarot Cards: The Beginners Guidebook To The Ancient Art Of Tarot Card Meanings And Spreads

Additional Reading

Complete Reflexology for Life Paperback – by Barbara Kunz

The Beginners Guide to Chakra's and Crystals Box Set:: A Beginners Guide To Crystals Their Uses And Healing Powers And Chakras

P.S. You'll find many more books like this and others under my name Michele Gilbert.

Don't miss them... here is a short list.

Introduction To Palmistry: The Ultimate Palm Reading Guide For Beginners

Emotional Intelligence: How to Succeed By Mastering Your Emotions And Raising Your IQ

Wicca: The Ultimate Beginners Guide For Witches and Warlocks: Learn Wicca Magic

The Introvert's Advantage: The Introverts Guide To Succeeding In An Extrovert World

Stop Playing Mind Games: How To Free Yourself Of Controlling And Manipulating Relationships

Instant Charisma: A Quick And Easy Guide To Talk, Impress, And Make Anyone Like You

Chakras: Understanding The 7 Main Chakras For Beginners: The Ultimate Guide To Chakra Mindfulness, Balance and Healing

Practicing Mindfulness: Living in the moment through Meditation: Everyday Habits and Rituals to help you achieve inner peace

Adrenal Fatigue: What Is Adrenal Fatigue Syndrome And How To Reset Your Diet And Your Life

Body Language 101: What A Person's Body Language Is Really Telling You...And How You Can Use It To Your Advantage

About Michele

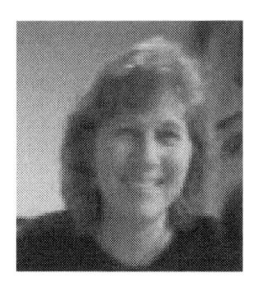

Michele Gilbert was born and raised in Brooklyn, New York. Drawn to literature and writing at a young age, she enrolled at Brooklyn College and majored in English. After graduation Michele did not begin writing immediately, instead she embarked on a career in the finance industry and spent the next thirty years on Wall Street.

Serendipity struck when she least expected it. After ending a long-term relationship, Michele found herself lost and unsure what the future held. She began to read books on grief and loss, looking for answers. Those led her to delve deeper into the Law of Attraction and its power. What resulted was remarkable. Not only had she begun to heal, she had also rekindled her former love of writing and discovered her life's purpose.

The years have taken her through many twists and turns, but she learned valuable lessons along the way. Today she publishes books-mostly self-help and metaphysical in nature-and feels compelled to share her knowledge with those facing similar experiences. Her greatest hope is to inspire others and show them ways to overcome adversity and gracefully accept life's inevitable low points.

Going forward, she plans to incorporate more teachings of self-help, finance and meditation. Regular meditation is very beneficial to her progress as she forges a new life. Morning rituals and positive incantations are other practices Michele embraces; they are very restorative in daily life.

As an avid hiker, Michele and fellow club members often hike the picturesque Jersey Pine Barrens. She is a history buff, voracious reader, baseball fanatic and a foodie. She also proudly supports Trout Unlimited-a national non-profit organization dedicated to conserving, protecting and restoring North America's Coldwater fisheries and their watersheds.

Michele currently resides forty minutes from Atlantic City and the Jersey Shore. She makes her home with a Blue Russian rescue cat named Jersey, though she isn't exactly sure who rescued who.

Michele really enjoys publishing books that can make a difference in people's lives. If you have any suggestions or would like to have a specific topic covered in a future book, please send an email to michelegilbertbooks@gmail.com and we will get back to you.

Thanks for reading!

Printed in Great Britain
by Amazon